"I read Dr. Bynum's bo[...]
ten it. I really like his use [...]
sense advice about taking [...]
life and health."

~*Dr. William Trumbower, M.D.*
Women's Health Associates, Inc.

"*Streaming Lifestyle: Healthier Living by Choice*" delivers practical yet motivational information that transcends the knowledge level of the reader. Those with a broad background in health and lifestyle theory will enjoy its easy, inspirational tone, while those with less knowledge will gain concrete insight and tips for better living. Dr. Bynum's way of conveying hope through visualizing a flowing stream is one to which we all can relate, while his personal story makes the journey seem manageable. We all need encouragement from time to time, and encouragement is what this book offers."

~*Deborah Barger MSN, RN,*
Certified Holistic Health Coach

"I was so pleased to see a medical doctor addressing wellness and prevention of illness through proper nutrition and hydration, stress reduction, physical activity and the belief system. All of the information was thought-provoking and simplified, which made it very empowering for someone who is searching for how to begin to take control of their own health.

It is encouraging to see Dr. Bynum stepping out of the western medicine tradition of treating symptoms with pharmaceuticals and empowering people with positive alternative therapies!"

~*Pamela Heyen,*
Certified Holistic Health Practitioner

Streaming Lifestyle:
Healthier Living by Choice

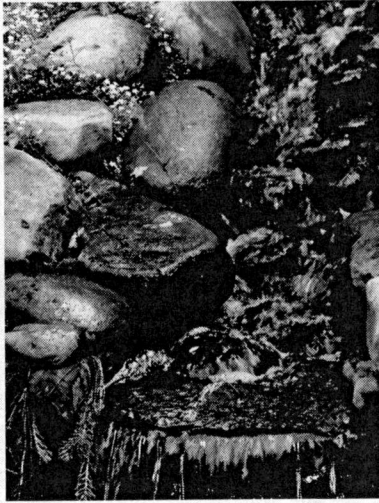

Dr. Robert L. Bynum
with Nancy Arant Williams

Lizm—
wish you the
best!
Be well &
Stream On!
Bob
2/14/13

© 2013 Robert L. Bynum
Streaming Lifestyle, L.L.C.

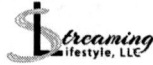

Writing assistance provided by
Nancy Arant Williams

Published by AKA-Publishing
Columbia, Missouri.

ISBN 978-1-936688-64-7

eBook ISBN 978-1-936688-65-4

Dedication

My brother, Bruce Bynum, had a passion for natural surroundings. He found that he was able to share this closeness to nature with his family by creating water features in the back yards of each of his homes. Pictured on the cover is the flowing stream at his most recent family home, completed just prior to his death.

His generous and creative spirit lives on in the memories and hearts of those who knew and loved him. This book is dedicated to him.

Acknowledgements

Each and every person throughout my life is part of my personal flowing stream, for it is the interactions with others that help create who we become. I appreciate the opportunity to realize the value each and every person has. You have the capacity to change another flowing stream in a positive way by paying it forward.

With that I want to acknowledge *you,* and hope that you find the will and way to encourage a positive change in yourself and others.

Many have touched this book in the making and I want to thank them all!

I want to extend my thanks to Lisa Bynum for providing water feature photos, and to all those who took time to read, provide feedback, and review the book.

A special note to Marty for planting the seed, Rachelle Kifer for being the ground to make it grow, Nancy and Yolanda for watering it, and my family, friends, and patients for being the sunshine!

Finally, thanks to the *Stream Team*—Deb, Tammy and Chris!

Your Streaming Lifestyle:
It's a choice

Try to imagine your body as a crystal clear stream high in the Colorado Rockies where the snow and ice begin to crack as they melt and begin a rapid downward descent. You can almost hear it now, can't you? And if you look closely you can see clear to the bottom of the stream bed, where there are rocks of all sizes, as well as a wide variety of plant life and colorful fish of every description.

The sound of a babbling brook is remarkably therapeutic—even comforting, isn't it? These days, people find it so appealing that they are building water features in their yards in record numbers, in order to relax and recover after increasingly stressful days at work.

With that word picture in mind, let me ask you a question: Has anyone ever told you that you're a walking miracle? A walking, talking, thinking human being—a phenomenon like no other? Well, it's true!

Just think of it—you are a one-of-a-kind individual, with DNA and fingerprints all your own. Your body is made up of billions of microscopic cells, each working in sync with the others, yet each one serving a very specific purpose. Like tiny, super-efficient factories, each cell is designed to function independently at peak performance, so that you can be the person you are meant to be. And like nearly all industrial processes, this feat requires a staggering amount of water to accomplish.

Human blood is actually made up of 92% water and delivers nutrients, enables cell function, removes toxins, and aids in repair and healing on a grand scale.

From the time we're able to choose for ourselves, it's up to us to decide what to do with our "stream." Over time, if we're not careful, it can fill with sharp rocks, accumulate sediment and debris, and ultimately lose its ability to flow freely. At that point it becomes slow-moving, somewhat stagnant, and not very appealing. As pollutants increase, the color changes from clear to murky brown, and the smell... well, you might want to think twice before drinking it.

Take a moment to consider this question: If I imagine my body as a stream, what does my stream look like? Is it crystal clear and free-flowing, or is it murky and slow-moving?

***

"I didn't think I needed to be humbled

but I guess God felt otherwise"

~ Dr. Robert L. Bynum

How this concept began

Perhaps this would be a good time to introduce myself. I am Dr. Robert Bynum, a practicing family physician for thirty years. I see patients in my office on a daily basis, and like to think of us—that is, my patients and I (and in this case you as well)—as team players in the health care process. Our greatest desire is to be well and flourish as we face the marvelous adventure we call life.

Like most other doctors, I've offered advice to patients over the years, suggesting things they could do to improve their overall health. And even if they didn't say a word, I could almost hear their responses in my head, and it wasn't a pretty sound. Of course, I didn't take it personally, because I've been there and don't like lectures (even cordial, compassionate ones) any more than the next guy. But while life changes are never easy, they are possible, and they really can improve our quality of life, even if we take baby steps on our way to our destination. The harsh reality is that doctors can't make anyone do anything, and I wouldn't want that to be part of my job description. I see my job as a kind of cheerleader, empowering you to do what works best for your particular situation.

Perhaps you've heard this definition of insanity: Expecting different results from the same old behaviors. It's true, but you can choose to participate in your own health care decisions, making changes that will ultimately benefit you more than you can even imagine. Your life stream is what you make it.

***

You know how they say that every doctor should become a patient at least once in his life, to understand how the other half lives? Well, that very thing happened, and after suffering a back injury, my focus changed dramatically. Since 2006 I have had two back surgeries, and the end result was debilitating chronic pain. As you can imagine, I certainly couldn't take narcotic pain medications and function with a clear head in the office. But what other options did I have? I say all this so you know I've been in that place where my "stream" was no longer free-flowing. I understand the frustration of being unable to move without pain, unable to continue living the kind of life I wanted.

Angry at the hand I had been dealt, I decided I was entirely too young to settle for that kind of life. That motivated me to search for other options, not just for myself, but for my patients as well. My life stream was literally screaming, demanding that I take charge to turn things around. Necessity—

or perhaps in this case, desperation—truly was the mother of invention.

Without making lifestyle changes, I tried multiple prescription medications. Unfortunately these did not work for me, either because of significant side effects or because they were ineffective.

After years of dealing with pain, I "got with the program." I went on an anti-inflammatory diet, lost 25% of my body weight, and started physical therapy as prescribed by my physician (and allowed by my insurance company). I continued to work out at home—walking or running on the treadmill almost daily. After all this, I experienced some improvement, but I still was not satisfied with the level of pain relief.

I started to do some new research and discovered supplements that addressed my pain and "stagnant flowing stream." After finding a new level of relief with these supplements, patients started asking me what I was doing and wondered if they could do the same thing. The quantity and expense of the supplements I was taking was more than most people were able or willing to afford, so I founded a nutritional company called ByPro Nutrition to manufacture quality products at a more affordable price.

My business partner suggested I write a book to tell my story, but after careful consideration, it seemed that presenting the "flowing stream" was much more important than my personal story. And thus this book was created.

Empowerment is the key

Over the years, patients have put doctors on pedestals, deferring to us as if we have all the answers, and to be perfectly honest, we've done little to change that perception. But the reality is that doctors are just human beings, products of our past and our education, and we all have preconceived notions and ideas that come into play when we treat our patients. Now that's not necessarily a bad thing, but it does tend to limit the choices given to patients.

This book was written to empower you to consider other options—to encourage you to think outside the box when making decisions regarding your personal health and well-being. The bottom line here is:

Don't allow others, even doctors, to make your decisions for you. The power belongs to you!

In the same way, people often assume that medications are the way to go for any and every ailment, especially because that's what the doctor recommends. What they may fail to understand is:

1) Through their personal experience, medical education, and possible liability issues, I believe many physicians carry a personal bias about alternative therapies, believing there are no other options than what they personally can provide. This also holds true on the other end of the spectrum, where those who believe in natural methods may see little to no value in traditional medical therapies.

2) Every prescription drug or supplement has potential side effects. What may work great for one person may cause severe and even life-threatening problems for another.

The other revelation I want to leave with you is this: Taking multiple prescription drugs and/or supplements only compounds the potential for negative drug interactions that can cause serious, irreversible health problems. So what's a person to do? For the sake of your life stream, you might research other options for the one that's right for you, because there may be many potential treatments out there.

Reputable sites on the Internet and the library are not the only available resources. Many health food stores and pharmacies have knowledgeable staff, and some even offer research libraries you can use to discover other options. Of course, you'll want to verify the validity of the information you read.

***

Insider information regarding prescription drugs:

Until the passage of the FDA Modern-ization Act of 1997, the Food and Drug Administration required drug companies to go through years of rigorous scientific testing to ensure that drugs were safe, effective, and pure before releasing them onto the market.

Pharmaceutical drug studies may be done on one specific group or population. Post-marketing results may show a different story or outcome regarding the effectiveness or associated adverse side effects of a product. Perhaps you've seen the television advertisements in which law firms invite you to call if you've suffered permanent ill effects from a prescription drug. Such issues arise as a result of dangerous drugs that were not stopped before they were released onto the market.

If you want to know about problems with a drug or procedure, research is the key. Correct information can empower you to make choices to help you protect your health and even save your life. The truth is that no one can protect your health and well-being the way you can, so you might want to be cautious about assuming a prescription drug is the answer to your problem when there are other available alternatives.

Insider information regarding statin drugs:

Researchers have found that sustained use of statin drugs, widely used to reduce cholesterol in the bloodstream, have a profoundly negative effect on levels of CoQ_{10}, a substance essential for efficient heart and cardiovascular function. Those who feel they must take statins may want to seriously consider taking CoQ_{10} supplements. However, in the grand scheme of things, a better alternative might be to simply watch the kind and quality of fats you eat.

Would you rather drink from

a flowing stream or

a stagnant pool of water?

Your body is mostly water.

Beginning your stream reconstruction

As remarkable as it sounds, no two life streams are alike, which means that as a one-of-a-kind individual, you deserve much better than a one-size-fits-all prescription for health. You need a customized program that fits your personal needs. You need someone who will listen to you, advocate for you, help you discover your options, and allow you to choose what works best for your stream. How does that sound?

***

To clarify things, it might help to have a little background on how the body works. Don't worry, there's no test at the end, just a hope that this process will make better sense once you understand what's really happening inside your body.

In the truest sense of the word, the human body actually consists of a vast series of complex microprocessors—everything is connected. All systems ultimately work in sync. Blood flows like a stream through blood vessels, sent on its way by a one-of-a-kind pump—the heart.

A remarkable organ, the heart begins to beat on the eighteenth day after conception, and pumps blood through a closed vascular system by the twenty-third day. It maintains this amazing pace at regular intervals, usually between sixty and eighty beats per minute, for the rest of your life.

It's difficult to fathom the number of times it will beat during your lifetime. At an average rate of sixty-five beats per minute, the human heart will have beat over 2.3 billion times by the time a person reaches seventy years of age. It's a stunning thought, isn't it? Though the heart is a relatively benign-looking organ about the size of a fist, I'm still struck with awe when I think about the longevity of this workhorse muscle.

The heart receives messages from the brain that tell it how much blood to pump depending on the body's activity level. When the body is relaxed or sleeping, it pumps just enough blood to supply the minimum amount of oxygen the body needs at rest. It pumps faster when the body is in motion, sending increased amounts of oxygen to all parts of the body.

Within the blood are red blood cells, ingeniously designed to carry oxygen from the lungs to all the tissues in the body as the blood makes its full circuit back to the heart. In addition to delivering oxygen and nutrients to feed the cells, the blood carries away carbon dioxide and waste within its winding stream. Its function is essential to every process in the amazingly efficient "factory" we call the body.

The heart starts out relatively light in weight. But after years of enduring stress, disease, mistreatment, and even malnourishment, it becomes heavier and cumbersome to carry. You may not notice any changes, but your body is well aware of what's happening. As your heart puts forth more effort to transport blood throughout the cardiovascular system, it also requires increased effort to take care of its own needs. It was a wise man who said, "If you take care of your heart, your heart will take care of you."

***

Metabolism refers to a set of chemical reactions that occur within the cells. It includes all chemical reactions that occur in the body, from digestion to the transport of blood, oxygen, and waste products through the body and from one cell to another. The efficiency of the metabolism is dramatically affected by how well our stream is functioning.

***

The nervous system impacts the body by sending and receiving signals that do many things, including calm the emotions, slow the heart rate and breathing, and ultimately reduce the amount of hormones the body needs. The opposite is also true if the stream is unable to flow freely.

***

The two components of the circulatory system—the cardiovascular and lymphatic systems—are truly the foundation of health. Through the circulatory functions, the body wards off illness and disease and keeps the organs and the body young, vital, and healthy. It is the system in which everything begins and ends.

In order for us to do our part to protect our streams, it's essential that we understand the cyclic nature of the circulatory system. Just as a river changes its course several times over its lifetime, the circulatory system makes adjustments in response to stress, illness, disease, and toxins.

The cardiovascular system is made up of a complex web of blood vessels including arteries (which primarily carry nutrients to the cells), veins (which transport waste and nutrient-depleted blood back to the heart), and capillaries (smaller vessels that aid in reaching all cells).

Veins, in particular, become less supple and elastic over time and benefit from good nutrition, supplements, and herbs in order to maintain their healthy, youthful function.

When the arteries are relaxed, blood flows more freely. When the body is relaxed, we notice higher levels of energy and a sharper mind, as well as supple, glowing skin. Sex organs are awakened, nerve endings are stimulated, and the brain sends a message to produce more pleasure hormones— otherwise known as endorphins—making our stream a happy place indeed.

The lymphatic system can be likened to the rocky bottom of a stream, filtering out toxins. This results in streams with clean, clear water flowing swiftly during high energy times, and flowing lazily during times of rest or relaxation. The lymphatic system is made up of lymphatic fluid, vessels, and lymph nodes, and is a vital part of the immune system.

Lymph nodes are tiny oval-shaped pouches that act as part of a dynamic filtration system. Located in various places throughout the body, they are connected by a network of lymphatic vessels. Loaded with white blood cells and macrophages, this finely tuned co-op works much like Pac-Man (of the bygone era video game), gobbling up enemies in its path. The job of these filters is to capture microscopic bacteria and viruses and destroy the unwelcome invaders before they can multiply and cause illness.

Unlike the cardiovascular system, the lymphatic system has no heart to pump lymphatic fluid from one place to another, which means there has to be another way. Guess what it is... Interestingly enough, we can help our bodies get rid of pathogens merely by staying physically active—simply getting up off the couch and moving around, doing our daily activities. I know it may sound implausible, so let me say that again. Being in motion, even ordinary motion, actually sends lymphatic fluid through the body to destroy disease-causing germs. Amazing!

Perhaps you've noticed tenderness and swelling in the glands on the sides of your neck beneath your chin when you have a sore throat or other infection—that's your lymph system in action. All in all, the lymph system works hard to keep our stream clean and free-flowing, with almost no extra effort at all.

Is your stream slowing down?

By the age of forty, the body makes less nitric oxide, a substance needed to signal the arteries to relax, and the powerhouse behind cardiovascular function. As we age, those levels decrease and circulation begins to grow sluggish. When people refer to "the normal aging process," they're usually referring to the need for increased nitric oxide. Poor circulation then sets off a cascade of effects, like dominos falling, making the victim feel far older than he really is.

Symptoms include: fatigue, mental fog, diminished sexual performance, increased blood pressure, slower wound healing, lifeless hair, and overall poor health. In time, a person will experience impaired range of motion in his muscles and be unable to accomplish things that used to be more or less effortless. At the point where even simple movement becomes painful and difficult, the person's self-worth takes a nose-dive.

Muscle atrophy and the accompanying impaired range of motion can be subtle at first and result from the aging process, a sedentary lifestyle, or circumstances beyond a person's control, but whatever the reason, it will have a profound effect physically, psychologically, and emotionally. At this point their life stream has a severely restricted flow that also has a domino effect, with each hindered system affecting the other. This causes the veins, which now struggle to open and close, to experience increased tension in order to compensate for the deficiency.

So what's the treatment for this malady? Increasing simple movement, regularly and often, can turn the situation around, raising nitric oxide levels before they reach the point of no return. With increased movement, blood flow and oxygen are once again restored to body systems. This increased movement not only improves resilience and nourishment to blood vessels, but also boosts brain and memory functions, increases energy level and stamina, and can enhance sexual performance.

In fact, we might even consider the body in motion a tried-and-true, inexpensive fountain of youth—another remarkable benefit for which our stream will thank us.

To go one step further, regular physical activity offers benefits that have no equal. As we have seen, increased movement encourages blood flow, which improves circulation and in turn ignites and maintains the immune system. The varied movements required in sports and other pleasurable physical activities offer incredible benefits to the body. And when physical activity includes movement that is out of the norm, it results in ever-increasing amounts of lymph to muscles and joints, so that in the end the body operates like a well-oiled machine, with increasing flexibility and strength.

Whether we want to believe it or not, the human body is made for movement, with joints, muscles, ligaments, tendons, and a skeletal system giving it form and shape as well as strength. We can go as far as to say that every body system is impacted by movement or the lack of it. Sitting for long periods of time can have an adverse effect on both the body's structure and its health.

The maxim, "Use it or lose it," has profound implications here. The reality is that what isn't used is eventually lost forever. Joints and muscles that are unused grow heavy, swollen, and weak and will soon lack the lubrication needed to move at all.

If we are wise, we will envision ourselves as "energy in motion." And a word to those with sedentary occupations: You can benefit by taking frequent breaks to bend, stretch, move, walk, and even lift hand weights to maintain flexibility and muscle tone.

When our stream's water grows precariously slow during sedentary periods, we risk being host to a stagnant pool, unable to regain movement necessary to cleanse the stream with the addition of water. Our bodies in motion open the underground spring that allows our stream to fill and once again flow freely.

***

Insider information about travel:

These days, people (especially retired baby boomers) have taken to the road in record numbers while they have the good health and finances to make it happen. However, they might want to keep in mind the importance of moving and staying hydrated, no matter what mode of travel they choose. Making it a point to stop, stretch, and move every hour, and drink adequate water, will help prevent blood clots and keep their life streams flowing exactly the way they were designed to.

Would you rather drink from

a clear mountain stream

or the muddy Mississippi?

Being your clean stream team

Keeping in mind that our bodies are over 60% water, let's take a look at fluid balance—that precision balance of water that keeps our streams functioning at peak performance.

Though we may have a beverage in hand at all times, if the glass does not contain water the majority of the time, we may mistakenly believe our fluid intake is sufficient when, in fact, we actually have a water deficit. Notice the distinction between the words "water" and "fluid." They are not the same thing.

We as human beings all have our favorite drinks, including but not limited to: fruit juices, teas, the ever-popular flavored coffees that now abound, soft drinks, milk, and the list goes on. But stop to think for a moment. Tea, coffee, and soft drinks usually contain significant amounts of caffeine that acts as a diuretic, leeching large amounts of fluid and releasing it through the kidneys. In effect, here's what happens: You can drink a gallon of liquids in total, but if that includes two or three cups of coffee, tea, or caffeinated soft drinks, the diuretic action pulls other fluids out with it, leaving your cells with a deficit instead of a credit in the fluid department.

Try this little experiment: For two consecutive days, keep track of what and how much you drink and how many times you urinate. On the first day, drink the fluids you would normally drink on any other given day. On the second day, consume only water and drinks without caffeine, and compare the difference between day one and day two. Then consider your life stream in this little equation. Perhaps it's time to pause and consider other options.

There are several symptoms that occur as a result of dehydration. One is brain fog, where you feel sleepy and struggle to complete a rational thought. Another symptom might be back pain or even a headache. If any of these symptoms occur, particularly after the noon hour, fill and drink a tall glass of cold, clear water, then wait twenty minutes and take note of how you feel. Something as simple as that can positively impact your life stream and performance both on the job and elsewhere—just something to keep in mind.

***

Insider information on soft drinks:

Medical studies have shown cola drinks containing phosphoric acid and caffeine to lower the bone marrow density (BMD) in the hip bones of women. X-rays tell the surprising tale: Those who drink copious amounts of cola display areas of bone deterioration and even holes, which allow the bones to fracture far more easily. Don't you just love insider information?

Nutritional choices and your stream

Maybe you've been confused over which foods to eat in order to lose weight and improve your overall health.

Well, first of all, let's take a closer look at the word "diet." It's been commonly used to describe weight loss formulas when, in reality, it just means what we eat. The word was actually never meant to be a verb, so perhaps it's time to toss it and begin thinking in terms of eating healthy and moving more in order to increase health and strength and maintain a healthy body weight.

So how can we feel and look our best? We can follow only our positive core beliefs, refusing to allow the negative to take hold, and then use wisdom to eat as healthy as we can.

At this point you may be asking, "What do you mean when you talk about core beliefs?"

Core beliefs are the things we believe about ourselves that affect every decision we make every day of our lives. They can be either negative or positive, depending on the kind of input we've had in the past and the things we tell ourselves. For instance, if my parents and other influential adults were kind and gave me confidence that I could accomplish whatever I set my mind to, my core beliefs would probably include the following: I am lovable, competent, gifted, able to master whatever challenge I face, I have options, I am capable of success, I fit in, I can change if I set my mind to it.

However, if my parents and other influential adults were cruel and demeaning, my core beliefs could look much different, and might include the following: I am incompetent, not good enough, unlovable, powerless, wrong, unwanted, unsuccessful, unworthy, a mistake.

With those two options in mind, answer this question: Do your core beliefs fall more toward the positive or the negative? Can you see how much they affect and color everything you do, every decision you make? While by nature some of us are more positive, we can each make it a personal goal to change the core beliefs that tend to tear us down. After all, who said we had to be perfect? If negative core beliefs, like sharp stones, are littering your stream bed, you can overcome them with your faith, meditation, daily affirmations, or by simply being mindful of them.

***

Now might also be the time to review the amount of sugars you are taking in through your choices of fluid intake. There are forty grams of sugar in a twelve ounce Coke, thirty-nine grams in a twelve ounce orange juice, and fifty-seven grams in a twelve ounce grape juice. While some of these sugars might be natural, too much of any good thing is like an algae bloom in your stream—not a desirable thing.

***

Insider information on eating healthy:

Simply eliminating processed foods and replacing them with fresh foods can make the difference in your energy level and your weight. Though it may not be obvious, both flour and sugar are recognized as sugar by the body. Starchy foods are merely chains of simple sugars, so watching your sugar intake means watching starchy carbohydrates too.

It might also be helpful to know that any food that is commercially packaged for mass appeal probably contains processed foods with little resemblance to what nature created. Here's an especially helpful hint: In order to shop healthier and eliminate the temptation of processed foods, try to limit your shopping to the outer perimeter of most grocery stores.

Insider information on food intake and sleep:

What we eat affects how we sleep. And to complicate matters, sleep deprivation can cause us to make poor food choices and tends to increase the desire to eat more empty calories. Several recent university studies have linked adequate sleep to the positive ability to take control of our health.

***

There are things you can do to improve your energy level, mental alertness, and even your sexual performance. Vitamins, supplements, herbs, and even the right prescription drugs can help you have a better life than you had previously, but the key is to step out of the box and decide what will work best for you. If you don't do it, who will? No matter what you choose to do, it's vital to protect your life stream in the process. Remember, it's going to be a lifestyle change over time, and not a quick fix that people often seek and never find.

A true lifestyle change involves embracing education to alter the way we think, act, and live, and addressing habits that are detrimental to our stream, all without compromising our positive core beliefs and what works best for our situation.

Getting healthy begins with "flow"—aiding the cardiovascular system, the lymphatic system, and the central nervous system so they operate at peak performance levels. Protecting and preserving our stream is the most important job we will ever have.

Insider information on weight loss:

As strange as it may seem, many people don't consider portion sizes when trying to lose weight. But when we take portion sizes seriously, we may find that we are actually eating double the number of calories we imagined. This is when reading labels can help. For instance, if the recommended serving size for oatmeal is a half-cup, then we either need to stop pouring when we reach the half-cup mark, or adjust our calorie count to include the amount we have poured. Sometimes we can be surprised by how small a half-cup serving really is. A good set of measuring cups can be invaluable to those who want to think realistically about portion sizes.

It can also help to use mindfulness— eating more slowly, savoring each bite, being aware of our intake, and realizing that it takes approximately twenty minutes for the stomach to notify the brain that we are no longer hungry. Keep in mind that it is never a good idea to eat when we are not hungry or are upset, even if that means we're eating out of sync with the rest of the world.

Which of the following lifestyles best describes the way you live? Niagara Falls, a rushing mountain stream, or a gentle babbling brook? Those who respond, "Niagara Falls," tend to move hard and fast, pushing themselves to the limit. Those who see themselves as mountain streams choose to enjoy moving at a brisk pace, but take fewer risks. Babbling brook people just want to move to stay healthy and feel their best.

No matter what your style, there are no limits to what you can accomplish except those you put on yourself. The key here is to follow through. We all make New Year's resolutions, most of which we never keep, but in this case, the choices we make to move our bodies will pay off bigger than a massive Powerball win. Really, what good is money if we don't have the good health to enjoy it?

Maybe you've heard this before, but it bears repeating here: How do you eat an elephant? One small bite at a time! The same thing applies to all major changes we plan to make in our lives. I might add that it's far easier to make a list of incremental small changes and check them off one at a time as we master them, than to try to conquer the entire project as a whole, which can often seem overwhelming or even impossible. Unfortunately, most of us quit trying when we get to that point, so it's important to take baby steps—establish positive new habits by repeating them over a six-week period, and then move on to the next thing on the list feeling excited and satisfied with a job well done.

Do you enjoy a leisurely walk in the evening or early morning? Do you just want some activity you can do in the privacy of your own home? Or are you competitive by nature, preferring to get out of the house and run a marathon, competing with others? The choice is yours, as long as you can envision yourself going there and doing it. Only you can prevent yourself from reaching your goals.

Insider information on regular physical activity:

It's important to incorporate an activity you truly enjoy if you are to keep it up for the long haul. It's also a great encouragement and often more fun to find a buddy who enjoys the same activity. The companionship helps with keeping your motivation up when you join forces.

Are you someone who started out at a consistent reasonable weight but gained over the years, so that you're constantly searching for the magic pill that will turn back the clock and make you slim again?

Well, consider this: If you do happen to get back to that ideal weight, you might not like the way you feel. Some people find that once they meet their goal, they feel weak and hungry, anxious and irritable all the time, which leaves them confused, wondering why. It happens because they no longer have the same metabolic needs they did when they were younger. If that's the case, they might want to ask themselves this question: At what weight do I feel my best and have the highest energy level, so that my life stream responds consistently with enthusiasm? Believe it or not, your mind and body will let you know.

Perhaps at age seventeen you weighed 125 pounds, and for years you've dreamed of getting back into those skinny jeans. Yet after an intense but moderately successful struggle to reach your target weight, it's still not working the way you imagined. Who says you have to get back into those jeans if you're happier, more comfortable, and feel your best at 160 pounds? Well, you may be asking, what about those actuarial charts the insurance people use that dictate my ideal weight? Don't tell anyone, but let's give ourselves permission to dump them in the trash where they belong, and do what works for us. Shall we?

Do you have smooth rocks

and let the water flow over them,

or do you have sharp, jagged rocks

cutting into your stream?

Stress and your stream

What about stress? Is it always a bad thing? Not necessarily. Even good things can introduce a certain amount of stress. It's how we handle it that causes problems.

For instance, the addition of a new baby is a dream come true for many young couples, and yet we've all heard the exhausted new parents (who feel as if the ordeal will never end) tell stories of sleepless nights and colicky infants. If we're in a position to do so, we can encourage them with the truth— it does end as the baby matures, and there are support networks, date nights, adult nap times, and hired baby sitters that can also help new parents weather the storm.

Even the dream job promotion—with increased pay and benefits—can cause stress due to the learning curve of new skills required to do the work. Whatever the blessing with its accompanying stressor, the key is to take things one day at a time, one step at a time, and understand that Rome wasn't built in a day. Be patient with yourself, recall the times in the past when you mastered new things, and know that you'll do it again.

These days, we've all seen businesses downsizing, and as hard as it is to imagine, our employers may be no exception. Long-term stress over even a rumor of potential layoffs can raise blood pressure, cause sleepless nights, and even result in stomach ulcers if our minds constantly jump to worst-case scenarios and we let worry consume our thoughts. So what's the answer to issues over which we seem to have little control?

First of all, it's good to once again pause and realize that *you are not your job.* You are a complex, talented individual born with creativity and imagination, as well as wisdom and common sense. If you are so moved, you might even lay out an alternative strategy just in case, and in the process let your inner child come out and play, thinking big. What would that be like? Well, consider this—many people who thought they would live and die in the same job have since been afforded new opportunities to ask themselves this question: What have I always wanted to do when I grew up that I never gave myself permission to pursue?

Many people are finding brand new life paths—new directions that work in concert with not only their life streams but their wildest dreams, bringing them new hope and great joy. If you could do anything your heart desires, what would it be? Really think about this.

One more thing about stress: It's here to stay, which is why we need to do all we can to adjust and cope with it. In the end, we must listen to what our bodies are telling us and respond accordingly.

Insider information on stress:

Stress can often be relieved through the practice of mindful meditation. By learning to detach ourselves emotionally from a stressful situation, we can train ourselves to observe and then respond (rather than react) to the difficult things around us.

***

You may be wondering: How does fear affect us? I'm glad you asked that question.

In some ways fear can be healthy, because it makes us use caution and wisdom in potentially risky situations. But we must take care that we don't allow fear to paralyze and hinder us from taking reasonable risks and stepping out to do new things we have the skills to accomplish. The thing to remember is to use due diligence, seek wisdom from those we respect who have lived longer than we have, and then take a moment to decide whether we'll regret not doing it in the end.

If the thought of a new endeavor keeps you up at night, excited by the prospect of the challenge, and you feel as if you can't live without trying it, it's probably right up your alley.

***

A behind-the-scenes look at stress and how it affects us: There are two types of stress that every person experiences on a daily basis.

Eustress is a positive type of stress that we often feel when faced with deadlines, challenges, and responsibilities that motivate us. It is best described as including feelings of anticipation, excitement, stimulation, enthusiasm, and passion. This good stress results in feelings of satisfaction with a job well done, a victory won. It inspires us to do better and work harder.

Acting on good stress through developing and carrying out a plan produces a sense of fulfillment and often results in others seeing us as high achievers capable of outstanding performance. If this describes you, it means you are doing what you love and succeeding at what you do because you give it everything you have to give. This kind of stress is essential to winning and succeeding in the challenges we face.

While you may never have heard the term "eustress" before, the second kind of stress is no doubt much more familiar. It's actually called "distress" and is the kind most people think of when they think of stress in their everyday lives. Distress causes negative responses such as anxiety, fatigue, depression, unhappiness, and even cardiovascular disease in the end.

Distress occurs when people are forced to function beyond their ability to perform, often doing things they hate. They have no time to relax when under duress—no place to stop and regroup. Their sleep may be disturbed, and they never seem to be able to rise above their circumstances. Feelings of doom and depression loom heavily over them until they eventually become physically, emotionally, and psychologically ill.

Such prolonged pressure can result in loss of hope, despondency, clinical depression, and eventually chronic feelings of despair if there is no end in sight. It can even block the positive impact of happiness and success so that nothing can penetrate the wall of negativity that is so firmly in place.

Negative stress can color the outlook so that everything appears in shades of gray, with no joy to be seen anywhere. At times it can be so overwhelming that it can shatter any possibility of future success.

The negative impact of stress can affect our life streams in the same way, making them resemble uncontrollable rushing rapids where water crashes over sharp rocks with enough force to change the color from clear to sudsy white. It moves so violently that it crushes rocks and reshapes the landscape without giving it a second thought. There is no denying that both distress and rushing rapids are destructive forces, yet if we can stay calm and look at things with a clear head, we can make lemonade out of the "lemon" situations in our lives, welcoming new life experiences and opportunities for creativity.

If we understand the two types of stress, we can be aware and prepared when we see the negative coming and take steps to address it before it consumes us. Once we equip ourselves with the facts, we can stop the downward spiral and examine our alternatives. Those in such situations can tell themselves the truth—they do have options and are not obligated to stay in distressing situations, no matter who says otherwise. Remember—the power is yours!

More about stress:
Modern life and new stresses

In our day and age, few people realize how much stress results from the constant barrage of noise and outside stimulation that our parents and grandparents never had to face. Most of them grew up in rural settings, wakened by the crow of a rooster, surrounded by birds singing in the trees.

Think about how much things have changed—we wake up to the stunning clamor of the alarm clock and spend every waking moment bombarded by light, movement, and sound, much of it loud and discordant. During a single half-hour café lunch break, you will no doubt see hurried people rushing about and hear the sounds of cell phones and other electronic devices bleating repeatedly, to say nothing of overhearing others' disjointed conversations wherever you go.

The electronic age may seem exciting, and despite the fact that many of us have embraced and even mastered much of it, in the end it can take a toll, causing great mental exhaustion. Ask most of those over age sixty, and they'll testify that they feel overwhelmed by sensory overload when they're out and about in today's world for any length of time.

The truth is that quiet is nothing to be feared; in fact, it might be considered therapeutic, a balm for the weary soul. Even for those of us who enjoy the relative chaos of our noisy, stimulating world, it might be a good idea to occasionally spend some time alone and in silence, giving thought to important things and being comfortable in our own company.

In the same way, information overload can cause unexpected stress. Email, television, radio, phones, iPods, Instant Messaging, Facebook, and Twitter, to name only a few, keep us constantly aware of news—some positive but much more of it negative, irrelevant, and unimportant—going on in our neighborhood and the world. How much news can a body take? If we find ourselves dreading the next message, we might want to consider turning off some of those "essential" devices.

Believe it or not, there was a time when people lived perfectly happy, contented lives without knowing what everyone else was doing, thinking, wearing, or watching every moment of every day. Reducing this kind of stress cuts down the demands on our adrenal glands, which respond with a powerful shot of epinephrine to help us cope when life gets to be more than we can handle.

The next question is: Do we even recognize the times when our lives become overly stressful and affect us in negative ways? It's certainly something to consider.

Do you suffer from hurry-sickness, always rushing, feeling pressured to do more in less time? If so, you may be missing out on the simple joys of life—beautiful sunrises and sunsets, picturesque scenery, and incredible people you may meet only once. Consider this: At the end of your life, you will be able to say one of two things—either, "I enjoyed my life, savoring every moment," or, "I wish I'd paid more attention to the beauty around me. I feel like it passed in a blur." We only live once, so let's not forget to stop and smell the roses. It will pay huge dividends for our life stream.

***

Insider information on stress:

One key to dealing with stress is to identify its source. Sometimes it's not obvious. But I recently learned that if you've become upset for no immediate or obvious reason, there's an underlying cause of some kind. When this occurs, ask yourself what it's about, and the source will often surface more easily than you think. If you can't readily discover the source of your stress, you may want to keep a journal of your daily activities, so you can go back and consider what effect they have on you.

Another clue: If you have any kind of nervous tic, be on the alert to what activates it. That precipitating event is definitely a stressor, from your body's point of view.

Insider information on N-Acetyl Cysteine:

N-Acetyl Cysteine is a nutritional supplement that has been shown to safely reduce anxiety and help people overcome depression, and can be especially useful when trying to break unhealthy habits such as smoking.

Something else to keep in mind: Your to-do list is never as important as your well-being while doing it.

Where do you locate your stream,

near a peaceful lush forest,

or a desolated desert environment?

Controlling your emotions

Emotions can greatly affect our life streams and have a tremendous impact on our health, which is why it's so important to evaluate what's going on in our hearts and minds when we're in turmoil. Sometimes the source is not what we think, but rather fear of loss of control, or even fear of failure.

Often we worry about what others think of us, when that really shouldn't factor into the equation at all. It's been said that what others think of us is none of our business, and perhaps this is often true.

Sometimes we allow others to offend us with offhand words or actions, but no matter who said what, it's up to us to choose how to respond.

Now, it's important to realize that some people feel empowered when they choose to hold a grudge and refuse to forgive others. But in reality they are only hurting themselves, because negative emotions cause chemical changes within the body and speed the process of aging and disease. Scientific research has shown that angry, discontented people are far more likely to die of heart attack and stroke than those whose outlook is positive and upbeat.

In the end, it is most healing to our minds to let go of offenses. Most people find it freeing to forgive, forget, or both! Cut the ties that bind and soar higher, with a clear mind and a clear conscience. Only a road block in your own mind can stop you from living your dreams.

In reality, few issues are worth the worry we give them; most work themselves out in the end with no action required on our part.

This is a good time to emphasize that we have the option to respond differently to stress than we have in the past. Oftentimes we tend to react with behaviors we automatically fall into when we feel that we have no options. In order to turn such feelings around, we can empower ourselves, telling ourselves the truth—that we do have choices, and we don't have to be knocked down by every negative thought that comes our way. When those kinds of thoughts come in to worry you and weigh you down, just tell them to leave, because they're not welcome anymore. Simply refuse to give them even one more second of your attention, and turn your focus to more positive things. Being proactive halts feelings of powerlessness and allows us to proceed without losing our objectivity.

Insider information on mindfulness and meditation:

Mindfulness is often learned through meditation practices, clearing the mind and enabling us to be thoughtful in our responses to life's everyday challenges. Meditation and prayer can help with renewal of the mind and increase your ability to accept that you can change. Each day is new and this is in itself an empowering thought. You may discover a new idea that will help you on your path to choices that lead to a healthier lifestyle.

It's healthy to have emotions, and it helps to know that sometimes just observing them and letting them go can be renewing. An important skill to learn is to respond thoughtfully to an event rather than simply react emotionally. Using mindfulness helps us make better emotional choices and can be a great tool in learning this empowering behavior. Respond or react—the choice is yours.

Perhaps you've noticed how the atmosphere can be affected by the kind of words and attitudes that are displayed in a given room. Oftentimes we enter a room with no clue of earlier conversation or events, but the tension is so thick that it's tangible, and if we're not on our toes we can automatically react to it with a fight-or-flight response (demonstrated by increased heart rate and blood pressure that occur when we start feeling uncomfortable). In that situation we can let go of it, realizing that it has nothing to do with us, then choose to respond with a smile, warmly greet others, and turn the atmosphere around. The power is yours!

It's true—laughter is the best medicine. Our bodies respond positively to humor, kindness, encouragement, affection, and affirmation, which is why we should freely offer these things at every opportunity, not only to others, but also to ourselves. I may only be one person, with a limited sphere of influence, but I am responsible to make it count for good, changing my little corner of the world and the one who dwells there—me!

Sometimes the world can be a harsh place to live, which is why it is said that we need ten positive affirmations to counteract every negative criticism. Often we can be our own worst enemies, refusing to forgive ourselves for our less-than-perfect performance. The thing is, life is tough enough without getting down on ourselves when we don't meet the mark. Responding to ourselves and others with kindness, learning to turn to our faith, and using mindfulness and affirmations will help us rise above the stresses of the daily grind and negative situations that arise. There are many styles of meditation being embraced in all faiths and in secular circles, and all are proven to help with clarity and coping skills. Our life stream will thank us repeatedly for such positive input.

In case that's not enough—have you heard it said that we each need an incredible ten hugs a day in order to be emotionally healthy? To be perfectly clear, this doesn't just include children. The sad truth is that few of us actually get that many, which just means we need to be gentle and give ourselves the equivalent of a hug whenever we need it. The little child inside us will certainly appreciate it.

Steering your stream

Sometimes people are overwhelmed even thinking about the word "exercise." The thought of a cardio workout twenty minutes a day, three times a week, can paralyze them and keep them from doing anything at all. If that's an issue for you, try thinking in terms of "activity" or "movement" instead. Sometimes just taking the pressure off by changing the language we use can eliminate the negative emotional connotation. As long as you make your life stream your priority, you will find yourself, more often than not, choosing to do the best things for your situation—a win-win every time!

***

Every day the body should be in motion from the time we wake until the time we go back into deep sleep. There are no guidelines to define what makes up a "normal" amount of movement, because we all move according to our own personal situations. The key here is to maximize whatever movement you do, making it count to keep your body fluid and flexible.

***

Remember this question: What would you rather drink from—a crystal-clear mountain stream, or the muddy Mississippi? A fast-flowing stream, or a stagnant pool? I assume you answered, "The mountain stream." In that case, let me give you a heads-up. As much as we might want to deny it, what we eat and drink matters. If we want our bodies to function, sparkling like a clear mountain spring, we will want to choose foods and drinks that will keep all systems go. If at all possible, we will want to buy organic produce, read labels, eliminate processed foods filled with chemicals, dyes, and preservatives, and drink plenty of good, clean (preferably filtered) water.

What we put in our mouths will affect our bodies and the way we feel, one way or another, so don't allow yourself to be lulled into thinking, "This doesn't count. It's only a little, and it can't hurt." It's that kind of long-term thinking that begins to tip the scale toward the muddy side of the equation. Instead of trying to straddle the edge of your boundaries, try asking yourself this question: What can I eat that I love that will also benefit my stream and help me feel my best? That's not to say we can never enjoy desserts and other things, but it's important to make those occasions rare and special, rather than an everyday part of our eating plan.

***

To be perfectly honest, I don't want to live by a strict set of rules every minute of every day, and you probably don't either. Overall,

I want to keep my body's best interests in mind, but I also enjoy a candy bar or a soft drink on occasion. The point here is to listen to your body, pay attention to what it's saying, and then try to maintain a balance between an anti-inflammatory diet and living on the muddy side. In the end, if I want to take control of my own pain and inflammation, I must make choices that produce the desired effect.

It may not be obvious, but inflammation is the underlying cause of most illness and disease, and it becomes far more evident as we age. When we keep inflammation to a minimum, we're actually paving the way for the body to function the way it was designed, even as we get older.

Insider information on inflammation:

Inflammation is the body's healing response to injury and infection. It works by sending immune cells and nutrients to the target areas. Sounds good, right? Well, consider this: Chronic inflammation that results from smoking, poor diet, stress, lack of sleep, lack of physical activity, and other immune system challenges can lead to chronic diseases like heart disease, diabetes, arthritis, and dementia.

***

We may not always be aware of how our food choices affect us, so let's look at the process: When we eat foods high in starch, sugar, and preservatives, foods with no nutritional value, the body rejects them and treats them like sediment that will not settle to the bottom of the stream. Because it has no place to use them, they continue to float in the bloodstream, hindering the free flow of blood. Foods high in man-made saturated fat and sugar eventually line the arteries with plaque, so that over time they become narrower and less elastic, further hindering the free flow of blood.

The heart, which is still responsible for pushing blood through the body, must now work harder to do its job. If this scenario isn't interrupted, the blood pressure rises to compensate for the extra effort of the heart. Inflammation builds at the site of the pressure build-up and results in pain—a warning that's hard to miss. If we fail to heed the body's warning that something is wrong, we miss our chance to turn things around. This is where we come in. When we can actually see the cause and effect of our actions, we can make changes that will transform how we feel and restore our ability to move as we once did, letting our streams once again sparkle and sing.

One of the first signs that the body has issues is lack of energy. By the way, it's also one of the most common reasons people see their doctors. It occurs when the body fails to get the nutrients and/or water necessary to do its job. It becomes especially frustrating when there is not enough energy to do simple daily activities. If the tide doesn't turn, you may then find that you need increasing amounts of sleep.

At the critical stage body systems begin to shut down, so that breathing becomes labored during normal activities—for instance, when walking across the room. The choices we make now will impact us either for good or for harm. Fortunately, our bodies are designed to heal themselves when given the right tools.

Insider information on mistaken beliefs of youth:

If you're not twenty anymore, you might recall thinking and even saying that you could do whatever you wanted, eat and drink whatever you wanted, and behave in whatever way you wanted and not be affected by it. Remember those days? Well, answer this question from your current viewpoint: Do you still believe those things?

***

Insider information on blood pressure:

You can lower your blood pressure with a hand grip. You know the one I mean—a steel coil between two handles. You hold it in one hand and squeeze hard for twenty seconds, then release and repeat for five repetitions with each hand. This process can relax the blood vessels and lower blood pressure without prescription drugs. (Note—at times, the blood pressure rises in response to sudden unusual situations that don't require long-term intervention. This can be the perfect time to use a hand grip.)

Another tip regarding blood pressure: You don't have to be a medical professional to keep track of your own blood pressure. In recent years, the process has been streamlined, and you can now buy a small, computerized wrist monitor with a digital readout that displays both blood pressure and pulse. It sells for under $40 and is available at most pharmacies and big box stores. It can allow you to stay in tune with what your body is saying and can be a great investment in your life stream!

***

I have a confession to make. I'm really no different than you. I've seen days so dark that I almost gave up on myself. Sometimes I'd rather drink a Coke than a glass of clear water. I even have occasional days when I crave potato chips and then eat the whole bag. However, I also recognize how my eating habits affect my body. As my system begins to age, I can actually feel an increase in pain and inflammation, and I notice I have far less energy. But as much as it hurts, it's a good thing—a signal that lets me know it's time to change direction in order to turn it around. None of us will be on target all the time, but the goal is to never give up. Being aware of what your body is saying will help you make wiser choices that will benefit your life stream. Remember, baby steps are still steps in the right direction!

***

Believe it or not, the foods we eat today are not of the same quality as those our grandparents ate. Today's foods are often grown in exhausted ground by hard-working farmers who must comply with the dictates of those who care far less about food value than the fact that the produce is bigger, brighter, and has more eye-appeal than ever before.

As a rule, farmland has been overworked and not allowed to lie fallow to recover and replenish exhausted nutrients and minerals. Large corporations, for whom the dollar is the bottom line, demand that every acre be planted every year, using the latest and most powerful chemical fertilizers, pesticides, and herbicides, so that the yield is off the charts. In order for farmers to produce the kind of crops these corporations demand, they must use more chemicals and grow crops using genetically engineered seed to produce even greater yield.

The only problem is that when we eat substances our body doesn't recognize as food, it can't readily break them down to use as nutrients and fuel. As a result, they remain in the digestive tract and the body reabsorbs them as toxins, not knowing what else to do with them. As toxins build up, they clog the circulatory system, significantly affecting the flow of our stream. A better option might be to buy organic foods at the local farmers' market, where quality produce came out of someone's garden.

Insider information on toxins:

Our bodies recognize aluminum, chlorine, and fluoride as toxic foreign substances that cannot be used. With no other options, these toxins collect in our tissues and muddy up our life streams, adding one more challenge for our already overworked body systems. You may be surprised to learn that we are often exposed to them on a daily basis.

In the case of chlorine, most cities add it to the city water supply to kill pathogens, which means that millions of people shower in it and drink it every day, with no idea that their tissues are storing up ever-increasing quantities of toxins. Those in this situation might want to consider installing a good water filtration system that will eliminate chlorine. That alone can enable the life stream to flow through a system unencumbered by toxic substances.

At this point, I want to emphasize the importance of reading labels. Believe it or not, many personal care products also include toxic substances. For instance, if you buy toothpaste at the grocery store, it probably contains fluoride. Ads have sung its praises for years, telling consumers that it protects teeth, particularly children's teeth, from cavities. But recent studies show that fluoride is a mineral that the body sees as a toxin, so it is important to refrain from swallowing it in order to prevent it from building up in the system and causing symptoms of toxicity.

**

Earlier we discussed how inflammation causes nearly all sickness and disease, so I thought it might be helpful to include a list of foods that inflame as well as a list of foods that heal. The lists that follow are only partial lists. Your own research may yield other information that is not included here.

Inflammatory foods list that can be found online using key words in your Internet search engine:

- Sugar
- Refined grains, white flour, white rice
- High fructose corn syrup (included in many packaged foods: read labels)
- Dairy products (consumed in excess)

Anti-inflammatory foods list by category, also found online using key words in your Internet search engine:

Fats:

- Extra virgin olive oil
- Avocado oil
- Salmon

- Sardines
- Herring
- Anchovies
- Flaxseed
- Hempseed
- Walnuts
- Almonds

Fruits & Vegetables:
- Onions
- Garlic
- Peppers, the hotter the better
- Dark, leafy green vegetables
- Cruciferous vegetables
- Apples
- Citrus fruits of all kinds

Herbs & Spices:
- Cinnamon
- Turmeric
- Oregano
- Rosemary
- Ginger
- Green tea
- Cayenne pepper

Protein:
· Grass-fed (not grain-fed) beef

Also available are diets designed to address specific health conditions. They are designed to omit certain offending foods that tend to aggravate the problem. If you have a chronic condition, you may want to research diets that address your particular condition.

Perhaps at this point you may be asking: What options do I have if I want to take control of my own health issues?

There are probably more alternative treatments than you ever imagined. The list includes but is not limited to (alphabetical):

· Acupressure and Acupuncture
· Aromatherapy
· Auriculotherapy
· Chiropractic
· Condition-specific diet modification
· Holistic Health Therapy

- Homeopathic medicine
- Lifestyle Health Coaching
- Massage therapy
- Physical therapy and activity, including aerobic and resistance conditioning
- Reflexology
- Vitamin and herbal therapy

A wide variety of books and articles are also available on these and many other treatment options. Research is the key to discovering which one will work best for you and your stream. In fact, you may opt to use a combination of several treatment options depending on your changing needs.

Let me say one last word here to encourage you to take charge of your future: You have only one life to live—one life to enjoy and make the most of—so don't let anyone talk you out of doing what works best for you and your stream. I'm rooting for you!

About the Author

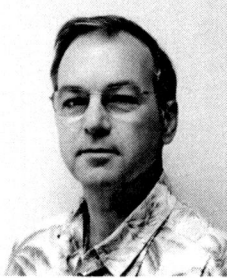

Bob Bynum, D.O., has been successful in family practice for over thirty years. Founder of ByPro Nutrition, he has formulated the nutritional supplements Dodecin® to reduce inflammation, and Triargin® to maximize body chemistry and promote optimum cellular function. Dr. Bynum also created the educational networking company, Streaming Lifestyle, LLC, which is dedicated to helping people find personalized options for developing healthier habits, making healthy choices, and living a happier, healthier life.

For more information on his philosophy and to find help changing your own direction, check out his website at:

www.streaminglifestyle.com.

CPSIA information can be obtained at www.ICGtesting.com
Printed in the USA
LVOW10s0859160813

348060LV00001B/1/P